The Menopause Chronicles

: Your Journey to Renewal

JOHN C.EXLEY

WELCOME TO "THE MENOPAUSE CHRONICLES: 5

CHAPTER ONE Fighting the Fire: Controlling Hot Flashes and Night Sweats..7

The Blaze's Nature 7

Equip Yourself with Information 8

Relief Techniques 8

Your Renewal Journey Continues 9

CHAPTER TWO Fighting the Fire: Controlling Hot Flashes and Night Sweats..10

The Fiery Onset..10

The Hormonal Offender 11

Appreciating the Process....................................13

CHAPTER THREE Embracing Hormone Harmony: Your Guide to Balance 15

Hormonal Symphony 15

Balance as a Lighthouse 16

The Nutritional Yin and Yang 16

CHAPTER FOUR: Mood Swings and Stress Management From Chaos to Calm...18

The Menopause's Emotional Landscape 18

Stress and Health...18

CHAPTER FIVE Reviving Your Libido: Rediscovering Intimacy 21

The Importance of Self-Care 22

CHAPTER SIX Food for Thought in Eating Well During Menopause 25

CHAPTER SEVEN 29

Exercise for a Vibrant You: The Power of Movement 29

    The Metamorphosis of Menopause 29

CHAPTER EIGHT 32

Mindful Moments: Cultivating Inner Peace...........................32

CHAPTER NINE 35

Sleeping Beauty's Secret: Conquering Insomnia 35

CHAPTER TEN Skin, Hair, and Self-Care: Beauty Beyond Age
....38

CHAPTER ELEVEN Rebirth and Renewal from Midlife to
Second Spring...42

CHAPTER TWELVE Wise Women's Wisdom: Stories of
Triumph and Transformation 45

Your Journey to Renewal," a transforming journey. Get
ready for an experience unlike any other, where the winds
of change whisper secrets of renewal, and the horizon of
midlife beckons with untold possibilities.

Menopause is not just an end but also a significant new
beginning and is frequently referred to as the unexplored
territory of a woman's life. Hormonal changes, emotional
peaks, and physical changes all come together in a
symphony. It serves as the entrance to your second spring,
which is full of life, insight, and self-awareness.

We shall examine the unsaid aspects of menopause in these
pages, those times when heat bursts like a phoenix's flame
and moods dance like erratically raging storms. On this
astonishing journey, we'll go beyond the obvious and the
clichés to reveal the extraordinary potential that lives
within you.

As you make your way through this change, get ready to
discover the secrets of harmony, beauty, and regeneration.
We will go into the art of accepting change, utilizing inner
strength, and learning from the past. It is a story of change,
where difficulties are overcome and you come out on top as
a brilliant, reborn phoenix rather than someone who has
been diminished.

Let the Menopause Chronicles serve as your inspiration,
reassurance, and direction. It's time to welcome this special
chapter of your life with open arms, confident that it offers

you the chance for regeneration and rediscovery. Your path to regeneration starts right now.

CHAPTER ONE
Fighting the Fire: Controlling Hot Flashes and Night Sweats

Consider this: You and your pals are having a pleasant talk, and there is plenty of laughter going on. Then suddenly, like an unexpected wave smashing on the shore, it hits you: a quick surge of heat that engulfs your body. It feels as though your whole essence has burned up as you are experiencing a heat flash.

Welcome to the sweltering world of hot flashes and nocturnal sweats, your unavoidable yet frequently vexatious menopausal companions. These erratic spikes in temperature have the power to transform a serene situation into a raging inferno. But don't worry; in this chapter, we'll provide you with the resources you need to douse the flames and regain your composure.

The Blaze's Nature

Let's first examine the fire's causes before trying to contain it. Hormonal changes, particularly the drop in estrogen levels that comes with menopause, are the cause of hot flashes and nocturnal sweats. Despite being one of the most prevalent menopausal symptoms, they vary widely. While some women just feel a slight warmth, others are subjected to intense heat.

Hot flashes affect more than just your physical health; they can also disrupt your routine, your sleep, and your general well-being. They serve as a reminder that your body is changing, but they do not have to dictate how you live.

Understanding the causes of hot flashes and night sweats gives you the capacity to properly manage them. We'll look at ways to reduce their frequency and intensity in this chapter. We'll look into the dietary considerations, relaxation techniques, and lifestyle decisions that can make a difference.

But keep in mind that you are not fighting this struggle alone. Many women have battled the menopausal embers and come out the other side stronger and wiser. You will find inspiration and hope in their experiences, which demonstrate that these difficulties can be overcome.

Relief Techniques

Let's now turn to reality. How do you put out the fire? We'll look at a variety of tactics, giving you a toolset to select from, ranging from natural cures and lifestyle changes to medical choices. Because each person's path through menopause is different, no one solution works for everyone.

We'll talk about the impact that diet and exercise play in controlling hot flashes, as well as how mindfulness and relaxation practices can help quell internal fires. We'll also look at complementary treatments and drugs for people who need more relief.

Even while hot flashes and nocturnal sweats are fearsome foes, they are not unbeatable. You can contain the blaze if you have knowledge, awareness, and a little bit of patience. These difficulties are merely stepping stones on your continuing route to rejuvenation and regaining your vigor.

Therefore, as we discuss methods for overcoming hot flashes and night sweats, keep in mind that you have the fortitude to face any challenge. Together, we'll forge a rejuvenated you from the ashes of menopause, transforming its heat into its warmth.

CHAPTER TWO
Fighting the Fire: Controlling Hot Flashes and Night Sweats

Many women are familiar with the feeling of an internal inferno that erupts without surprise during menopause, leaving you hot, sweating, and searching for respite as you navigate the frequently choppy sea of hormonal shifts.

Welcome to the realm of night sweats and hot flashes, when putting out the fire becomes a major plot point in your Menopause Chronicles.

The Fiery Onset

The majority of women who experience menopause experience hot flashes and nocturnal sweats as it is a changing time in their lives.

Whether you're quietly dozing off in the middle of the night or the middle of a business meeting, these unexpected heat waves can occur at any time.

Hot flashes include The sudden, strong feeling of heat that characterizes these daily episodes and is frequently accompanied by skin flushing, a quick heartbeat, and profuse sweating.

They could persist for several minutes or only a few seconds.

Night sweats are essentially heat flashes that happen while you're sleeping. They might wake you awake, leaving you bathed in perspiration and frantically searching for the cool side of the pillow.

We must first identify the hormonal causes of these ferocious outbursts to comprehend how to control them.

The changing estrogen levels that come with menopause are a major cause of hot flashes and nocturnal sweats.

The hypothalamus, a part of the brain that controls body heat, is influenced by estrogen, a critical role in controlling body temperature.

The hypothalamus becomes more sensitive to temperature variations when estrogen levels fall, causing it to interpret even little shifts as large heat surges. The outcome? Your body's thermostat malfunctions, resulting in those jarring, scalding hot flashes.

The Effect on Daily Life
Hot flashes and nocturnal sweats can significantly affect how you live your life. They may interfere with your sleep, work, and social life, making it difficult for you to concentrate and making you feel worn out. These outbursts can sometimes be followed by emotions of irritation or humiliation, which adds to their emotional burden.

The Battle Techniques

Now that we know who the ferocious enemy is, let's look at some combat tactics to subdue hot flashes and night sweats:

1. Keep Cool: Dress in layers, choose breathable materials, and maintain a comfortable temperature in your home. Air conditioning or using fans might also be beneficial.

2. Deep, diaphragmatic breathing exercises can assist your body in responding to heat flashes by lowering body temperature. To relax your body, try tactics like taking slow, deep breaths.

3. Maintain Hydration: Drink plenty of water throughout the day since dehydration can make hot flashes worse.

4. Track Triggers: - Keep a journal to note down the particular situations that set off your hot flashes. Spicy foods, caffeine, alcohol, and stress are typical offenders.

5. Herbal Treatments: - Some women get relief from hot flashes and night sweats by using herbal supplements like evening primrose oil or black cohosh. Before beginning any new supplements, speak with your healthcare provider.

6. Prescription Alternatives: Your healthcare practitioner can advise hormone replacement therapy (HRT) or other prescription drugs for severe symptoms that have a major impact on your quality of life. These need to be thoroughly discussed, taking into account any dangers and advantages.

Hot flushes and night sweats may seem like powerful foes, but they also serve as a tribute to your body's adaptability and tenacity.

They represent the significant internal changes you are going through as you enter menopause. Accepting this road and all of its difficulties might result in personal development and transformation.

Getting Assistance

Keep in mind that you are not fighting this war alone. Ask for advice from friends, relatives, or support groups by reaching out to them.

Sharing experiences and tactics can frequently offer both emotional support and workable solutions.

The Renewal of Things Beyond

Remember that this chapter of your Menopause Chronicles is just one portion of a larger adventure as you travel over the turbulent seas of hot flashes and nocturnal sweats. Menopause's fires may burn, but they also show us the way to renewal.

You are encouraged to go into the depths of your strength, flexibility, and resilience during this period.

May you discover the ability to withstand the fire as you fight it and come out the other side stronger and more in control than before.

The chapters that follow will go into greater detail about this life-changing journey, examining techniques for controlling mood swings, embracing hormone equilibrium, and rekindling desire.

These are the factors that mold your path to rejuvenation and serve as a gentle reminder that menopause is not just a struggle to get through but also a fascinating and empowering chapter in your life narrative.

CHAPTER THREE
Embracing Hormone Harmony: Your Guide to Balance

Imagine this: A captivating dance in the air is produced by a mobile that is properly balanced, with each component suspended in harmony.

Imagine your body as that mobile system right now, with hormones acting as the fine strings that keep everything in place.

Menopause upsets this delicate balance for many women, causing hormones to undergo a rapid transition.

But don't worry; in this chapter, we'll examine how to achieve hormone harmony amid the confusion.

Hormonal Symphony

The unheralded conductors of your body's orchestra, hormones control everything from your metabolism and mood to your sleep and sexual desire.

However, they appear to rebel throughout menopause, leading to emotional peaks and physical discord. It sounds like the orchestra is playing a strange piece.

The key to navigating the menopausal journey is to comprehend this symphony. Once abundant, estrogen, progesterone, and testosterone now play different roles as they become less prevalent.

Mood swings to alterations in bone density are just a few

of the symptoms that might result from these hormone shifts.

Balance as a Lighthouse

The key to tuning an instrument amid this hormonal symphony is finding equilibrium. The music flows easily when the strings are in tune. Similarly, you feel healthy and energetic when your hormones are in balance.

But what exactly does a hormonal balance entail? The goal is to control the oscillations rather than eliminate them. It involves accepting the ups and downs of menopause while minimizing its more difficult parts. This equilibrium demands a diverse strategy to achieve.

The Nutritional Yin and Yang

Nutrition is one of the most efficient strategies to restore hormone balance. Your diet has the power to either quell the menopausal fires or ignite the flames of imbalance.

In this chapter, we'll examine the effectiveness of a diet full of phytoestrogens, antioxidants, and necessary nutrients for menopausal sufferers. You'll learn how some foods can help with hormone balance, symptom relief, and general well-being.

The Dance of Physical Activity and Relaxation

The restoration of equilibrium also heavily relies on exercise and relaxation methods.

Regular exercise not only keeps your body fit but can also aid with hormone regulation and mood enhancement. On the other hand, relaxing techniques like mindfulness and meditation offer relief from the emotional upheaval that is frequently connected to menopause.

Your Road to Renewal
Always keep in mind that this journey is about you as we continue to explore the art of embracing hormone harmony.

It's about figuring out what suits your particular physique and situation the best. Even amid the menopausal tumult, your life's mobile can restore equilibrium and begin to dance to lovely music once more.

You will be directed in this chapter toward tactics and routines that support hormonal balance. It's a trip toward rejuvenation, a journey toward recovering the equilibrium that, although it may have appeared elusive, is very much within your grasp.

So let's start this peaceful journey together, dear reader, and accept that your hormonal ebbs and flows are a necessary part of your change.

By doing this, you'll discover the menopause's rhythm and learn to use it to create a fresh, lively symphony of life.

CHAPTER FOUR:
Mood Swings and Stress Management From Chaos to Calm

Imagine waking up and being on an emotional whirlwind. You can be on cloud nine one second and then sink into the pit of despair the next.

Welcome to the world of menopause's mood swings, a rollercoaster of feelings that can make you feel out of control. But do not worry; in this chapter, we will discuss how to achieve tranquility within the turbulence and turn this chaos into quiet.

The Menopause's Emotional Landscape

Menopause mood swings are like unexpected storms that sweep in and leave you drenched in frustration, despair, or even wrath. Although these emotional changes might be confusing and lonely, they are a normal aspect of the menopausal experience.

Your mood may be impacted by the hormonal changes associated with menopause, which may disturb the delicate balance of neurotransmitters in your brain. The mood-regulating hormone estrogen plummets, which frequently results in feelings of anger and melancholy.

Stress and Health

Stress and mood swings frequently go hand in hand. Stress can be amplified by the pressures of daily life as well as the menopausal physical and emotional changes.

A difficult feedback loop results from stress aggravating mood changes.

We'll examine the complex connection between stress and mood fluctuations in this chapter. You'll learn how persistent stress affects your body, psyche, and symptoms of menopause.

But more significantly, we'll give you the tools you need to end this vicious cycle and find serenity amid the mayhem.

Emotional Resilience Tools
The first step on the path from chaos to tranquility is self-awareness. The first step is to recognize the patterns and factors that cause your mood fluctuations.

After that, we'll look at useful strategies and methods that can assist you in regaining emotional equilibrium.

We'll delve into mindfulness techniques that help you stay in the present and offer refuge from the storm of emotions. Additionally, you'll learn the effectiveness of deep breathing techniques, which can calm your nervous system and lessen the severity of mood swings.

Seeking Assistance
On this emotional journey, you're not going it alone. Friends, family, or support networks can be a tremendous help.

Sharing your thoughts and feelings with people who can

relate to what you're going through might help you feel less alone and more at ease.

Another helpful tool is seeking out professional assistance, such as through therapy or counseling. Therapists can provide you with the coping mechanisms you need to deal with stress and mood swings, enabling you to move through this difficult terrain with grace and resiliency.

The Road to Inner Peace
Keep in mind that this chapter is a guide to discovering inner calm as we negotiate the terrain of mood swings and tension.

Although your emotions may fluctuate, you can guide your emotional ship through a storm.

You don't have to let the craziness of menopausal mood swings define your path. Instead, use it as a springboard for change, a chance to learn more about yourself, and a stride towards the serenity that is just ahead.

So let's begin this journey from turmoil to serenity together, dear reader, armed with wisdom, comprehension, and a steadfast dedication to your mental health.

Your path to regeneration includes finding calm amidst the chaos, and it starts right here.

CHAPTER FIVE
Reviving Your Libido: Rediscovering Intimacy

Close your eyes and recall a period when love flowed naturally, intimacy was an adventure, and desire surged like a wild torrent. Imagine if those times are now in the future rather than in the past. Welcome to your journey's chapter where we examine how menopause might act as a catalyst for finding your libido and rekindling the flames of connection.

The Labyrinth of Libido
Your libido—the ember of desire and intimacy—can be impacted by the changes that menopause frequently brings about in your body and emotions.

But keep in mind that these alterations represent a fresh start rather than a conclusion.

It is crucial to comprehend the complex relationship between hormones, emotions, and intimacy. Sexual desire may be affected by vaginal dryness and discomfort brought on by the decline in estrogen.

You may not be as interested in intimacy if you are experiencing emotional changes, such as stress or mood swings. However, there is light at the end of this maze.

Communication Is Crucial

With a partner, navigating this terrain demands direct and honest communication. Your partner can be an invaluable ally and source of support on your journey to rejuvenation.

Your relationship can be strengthened and a safe space for intimacy to grow by talking about your needs, worries, and boundaries. Encourage open communication and understanding among all parties before starting this adventure.

Accepting Change

You are encouraged by menopause to accept change, including a change in how you view intimacy.

It's an opportunity to investigate novel facets of pleasure, one that emphasizes shared experiences, communication, and emotional ties.

We'll look at how you might adjust to these changes and discover new avenues for closeness in this chapter.

It's an opportunity to rewrite the story and learn that closeness is not constrained by advancing age or bodily changes.

It has the potential to develop and deepen, fostering fresh connections and pleasure.

The Importance of Self-Care

Self-care is also a part of reviving your libido and rediscovering connections. Maintaining your physical and mental health is an investment in your close relationships.

In addition to addressing common menopausal issues like vaginal dryness and soreness, we'll talk about stress management and mood stabilization tactics that might affect your desire.

Broadening Your Perspectives
Your quest for rebirth entails discovering fresh realms of pleasure and closeness. We'll talk about how to rekindle your passion and how to practice mindfulness, self-discovery, and sensory experiences.

Stories of women who changed their romantic lives during menopause will inspire you and show you that desire has no age restrictions.

Your Journey Goes On
Your sense of intimacy and desire are fundamental components of who you are, and menopause need not lessen them.

It might be the spark that rekindles your libido and helps you rediscover the depths of intimacy.

Keep in mind that this chapter of your trip is one of exploration and rediscovery as you set out on it. It's a chance to connect with your desires, be honest with your relationship, and put self-care first.

Your libido is a dynamic energy that can burn even hotter in this stage of life; it is not a relic of the past.

So let's go down this road of rediscovery together, dear reader. May you realize that the flames of desire burn brighter and more fiercely than ever as you rekindle your libido and rediscover intimacy?

CHAPTER SIX
Food for Thought in Eating Well During Menopause

Think of your body as a beautiful garden. Its growth and blooming are influenced by the food you give it. It's more important than ever to care for your garden as you negotiate the complex landscape of menopause. In this chapter, we'll look at how the correct meals can help you along the way by giving you the energy and nutrition you need to thrive.

The Menu for Menopause

The menopause is a time of transition, and your body's nutritional requirements may change at the same time. Hormonal changes can have an impact on your metabolism, bone health, and general wellness.

Your move through this transformative phase might be helped or hampered by the foods you select.

Let's start with comprehending the fundamental elements of a diet that is menopause-friendly:

1. *Foods including soy, flaxseeds, and legumes have substances that mimic estrogen in the body, potentially lessening menopausal symptoms. This is known as phytoestrogens.*

2. *Vitamin D and calcium: During menopause, these nutrients are essential for preserving bone health. Leafy greens, dairy products, and fortified foods are all great sources.*

3. *Omega-3 Fatty Acids: These fats, which are present in fatty fish, flaxseeds, and walnuts, can reduce mood fluctuations and promote heart health.*

4. *Foods High in Antioxidants: Oxidative stress that may be brought on by menopause can be reduced by eating a diet high in colorful fruits and vegetables.*

5. *Hydration: Maintaining a healthy level of hydration is important since it can help with symptoms like hot flashes.*

Portion Control: An Art

It's important to consider both what you eat and how much when you go through menopause. Portion management is a useful skill during this phase because metabolism tends to slow down.

Eating consciously and paying attention to your hunger cues can help you maintain a healthy weight and prevent unintended weight gain, which is frequently linked to menopause.

A Balanced Strategy

The fact that there is no one-size-fits-all diet for menopause must be emphasized. Your path through this phase is unique, as are your nutritional demands. The goal is to maintain portion control, balance your diet with the

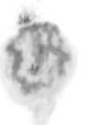

appropriate nutrients, and pay attention to how your body is changing over time.

Getting Around Dietary Obstacles

Dietary concerns related to menopause may include controlling weight, treating digestive problems, or accommodating food sensitivities.

We'll offer advice on how to deal with these difficulties and make wise decisions in this chapter.

Enjoying the Travel

Maintaining a healthy diet throughout menopause is not a burden; rather, it is a chance to enjoy the trip.

It involves learning about scrumptious, wholesome foods that promote your well-being. It's about enjoying yourself in the kitchen and taking good care of your body.

Keep in mind as you read through this chapter that part of your path to regeneration includes feeding your body from the inside out.

Food is a source of vigor and wellness in addition to providing sustenance. It's a crucial aspect of your menopausal journey, and making the proper decisions can provide you the strength to thrive at this pivotal time.

So let's start this culinary journey together, my reader. May your journey as you embrace the art of eating well through menopause be full of delectable discoveries, rekindled vitality, and the delight of tending to your lovely garden of well-being.

CHAPTER SEVEN
Exercise for a Vibrant You: The Power of Movement

Imagine feeling your body moving, your heartbeat synchronized with each step or stretch. This is the power of movement—a tonic for your mental and emotional health as well as a crucial ally during menopause. This chapter will examine how exercise may change your life and how it can make it more vibrant.

The Metamorphosis of Menopause

Your body goes through the menopause, which causes changes to your metabolism and muscle mass. Physical activity now is not only helpful but also essential. During this transformational stage, exercise can improve your overall health by reducing the consequences of hormone swings.

The Advantages Outside the Body

Exercise has many benefits outside of just physical health. Regular physical activity can work as a powerful mood stabilizer and stress reliever.

It can also improve your mental wellbeing. It's a mental reset that can lift the menopausal-related brain fog that's so common.

Discovering Your Movement Joy

Exercise is wonderful because it is such a very personal experience. It involves identifying the pursuits that connect with you, make you happy, and make you feel alive.

 Any activity that gets your body moving and your soul soars qualifies, whether it be dancing, hiking, yoga, swimming, or anything else.

We'll assist you in this chapter as you investigate numerous forms of exercise to determine which ones best suit your preferences and way of life.

We'll talk about the importance of strength training for preserving bone and muscle mass as well as the advantages of aerobic exercise for strength and endurance.

The Benefits of Mindful Movement
Exercise can benefit from mindfulness, which is the art of being present in the moment. Moving mindfully may improve your relationship with your body, ease stress, and maximize the health advantages of exercise.

Overcoming Obstacles
We'll also talk about typical obstacles women encounter when trying to exercise during menopause. We'll offer tips to get beyond these roadblocks so that exercise becomes a regular and joyful part of your life, regardless of whether they are caused by a lack of time, a lack of enthusiasm, or physical difficulties.

The Journey Goes On

Exercise is a continuous journey of self-discovery and regeneration; it is not a destination.

You'll learn that harnessing the power of movement is about more than simply physical change; it's also about restoring your vigor, your strength, and your sense of self.

So let's start this chapter of your adventure together, dear reader. May you experience the vivacious energy pulsing through your veins, energizing your body and reviving your spirit, as you harness the power of movement, with each step, stretch, and moment of movement, the road to regeneration is paved.

CHAPTER EIGHT
Mindful Moments: Cultivating Inner Peace

Close your eyes and take a deep breath. Feel the gentle rise and fall of your chest, the sensation of the air filling your lungs. At this moment, you're practicing mindfulness—a powerful tool for finding serenity amidst the whirlwind of menopause. In this chapter, we'll explore the art of cultivating inner peace through mindfulness, inviting you to embrace the present and discover a sanctuary within.

The Menopausal Maze

Menopause often feels like navigating a labyrinth, with unexpected turns and emotional twists. The hormonal fluctuations and physical changes can leave you feeling like a passenger on a rollercoaster. But within this maze lies the opportunity for self-discovery and renewal.

The Gift of Mindfulness

Mindfulness is the practice of being fully present in the moment, without judgment. It's a profound gift you can give yourself during menopause—a gift that allows you to step off the rollercoaster and find solid ground.

When you practice mindfulness, you become an observer of your thoughts and emotions. You learn to acknowledge them without attachment or judgment, allowing them to flow through you like clouds in the sky. This practice empowers you to respond to menopausal challenges with clarity and composure.

The Mind-Body Connection

Menopause is not just a physical transition; it's a deeply interconnected mind-body experience.

Mindfulness can bridge this connection, offering relief from the emotional turmoil that often accompanies menopause symptoms.

We'll explore how mindfulness techniques can alleviate mood swings, reduce stress, and improve your overall emotional well-being.

By integrating mindfulness into your daily life, you can transform menopausal challenges into opportunities for growth and self-compassion.

Cultivating Mindfulness

In this chapter, we'll guide you through various mindfulness practices tailored to the unique challenges of menopause.

You'll learn techniques for managing hot flashes, soothing anxiety, and improving sleep quality. We'll also delve into mindfulness-based stress reduction (MBSR) practices,

which are effective in enhancing emotional resilience during menopause.

Mindful Moments

Mindfulness is not just a practice; it's a way of life. We'll discuss how you can infuse mindfulness into your daily routine, creating moments of serenity and self-compassion. Whether it's through meditation, mindful eating, or simply pausing to savor the present, you'll discover that mindfulness can be your trusted companion on this journey.

Your Sanctuary Within
As you embark on this chapter of your journey, remember that the path to renewal lies within you.

Mindfulness is the key that unlocks the door to your inner sanctuary—a place of peace, resilience, and self-discovery.

It's a journey of nurturing your mind and spirit, just as you nurture your body.

So, dear reader, let's embark on this mindfulness journey together. As you cultivate inner peace and embrace the present moment, may you find solace during change, strength in the face of challenges, and renewal in every mindful breath you take.

CHAPTER NINE
Sleeping Beauty's Secret: Conquering Insomnia

Imagine a night when you slip effortlessly into slumber, your body and mind cradled in the comforting embrace of sleep. Your journey through menopause, however, might have disrupted this peaceful reverie with the unwelcome guest of insomnia. In this chapter, we'll explore the secrets to conquering insomnia and unlocking the restorative power of sleep.

The Nighttime Struggle

Insomnia is a common companion during menopause, and it can feel like a relentless foe. The hormonal changes, hot flashes, and mood swings can create the perfect storm for disrupted sleep. But fear not, for strategies and secrets can help you regain control of your nights.

The Importance of Sleep

Sleep is not merely a luxury; it's a vital component of your physical and emotional well-being. It's during sleep that your body repairs itself, your mind processes the events of the day, and your emotions find equilibrium. Quality sleep is the key to waking up refreshed and ready to embrace each day.

The Sleep-Deprived Menopause Cycle

Insomnia can create a vicious cycle. Sleepless nights lead to increased stress, mood swings, and fatigue, which can, in turn, exacerbate insomnia. It's crucial to break this cycle and prioritize sleep as a cornerstone of your menopausal renewal.

Unveiling the Secrets
In this chapter, we'll unveil the secrets to conquering insomnia and restoring restful sleep. These secrets include:

   1.   Sleep Hygiene:
  - Learn the art of creating a sleep-friendly environment, from optimizing your bedroom to establishing a calming bedtime routine.

   2.   Stress Reduction:
  - Explore techniques for managing stress and anxiety, as they are common culprits behind insomnia.

   3.   Nutrition:
  - Discover how dietary choices can impact your sleep patterns and what foods can support restful sleep.

   4.   Herbal Remedies:
  - Explore natural remedies, like herbal teas and supplements, that can promote relaxation and sleep.

   5.   Mindfulness:
  - Integrate mindfulness practices into your evenings to quiet a racing mind and prepare for rest.

   6.   Medical Solutions:

- Understand when seeking medical intervention for severe insomnia may be appropriate and discuss potential treatment options with your healthcare provider.

Your Path to Renewal

Conquering insomnia is a vital step on your journey to renewal. It's about recognizing the importance of sleep and taking proactive steps to restore your body's natural rhythm.

It's about embracing the secrets to restful sleep and making them a part of your daily life.

So, dear reader, let's embark on this chapter of your journey together. As you unveil the secrets to conquering insomnia and rediscover the restorative power of sleep, may you awaken each day feeling refreshed, renewed, and ready to embrace the possibilities that lie ahead.

Sleep is your ally in this journey, and its secrets are your key to a brighter, more vibrant tomorrow.

CHAPTER TEN
Skin, Hair, and Self-Care: Beauty Beyond Age

Imagine looking in the mirror and observing not only the changes brought about by time but also the beauty that results from knowledge and experience. In this chapter, we'll look at how to embrace aging with grace and confidence by taking good care of your skin, hair, and other body parts during menopause.

The Aging Canvas

Menopause is a moment of transformation, and its consequences extend outside of your own space. In line with changes in your hormones and metabolism, your skin and hair also alter.

But keep in mind that these changes are a natural part of becoming older and can be welcomed as a part of your journey.

Caring For Your Skin

Your skin is a window into the health and happiness of your soul. It could become drier, thinner, and more prone to wrinkles throughout menopause.

However, these modifications are not permanent. You can hydrate your skin and replenish its vitality with the proper treatment.

We'll talk about menopausal-specific skincare regimens in this chapter. You'll learn the value of skincare products that support collagen and elasticity development, hydration, and sun protection.

We'll also discuss all-natural cures and treatments that help improve the health and shine of your skin.

Adore Your Hair
Your hair is an additional canvas on which the art of aging takes shape. You could notice variations in the texture and color as it gets thinner.

However, you should embrace these changes since they make you wholly beautiful.

We'll talk about hair care regimens that are tailored to the unique requirements of menopausal hair. You'll discover how to pick the best products, deal with hair loss issues, and adopt looks that enhance your inborn beauty.

Ritualizing Self-Care
Self-care is an essential discipline for nourishing your body and spirit; it is not a luxury. Self-care should become a daily practice during menopause as a way to honor your body and mind.

We'll examine the practice of self-care in this chapter, which includes activities like:

1. Mindfulness: - Methods for increasing self-compassion and lowering stress, which are good for your skin and general health.

2. Nutritional Support for Healthy Skin, Hair, and Nails: Foods and Supplements.

3. Exercise: - How moving about can increase circulation, which promotes healthier skin and hair.

4. Sleep: - Making healthy sleep a top priority as an integral part of self-care.

5. Emotional Well-Being: - Techniques to increase your self-confidence and self-esteem while you deal with the changes brought on by menopause.

Your Journey

As you begin this chapter of your journey, keep in mind that beauty is not just for young people. It is ageless, and every stage of life has its special allure.

Your skin, hair, and self-care are all components of the painting that depict your experiences and personal development.

Accept the practice of caring for your skin, hair, and body as an expression of self-love. Celebrate your inner brightness and the beauty that exists regardless of your age.

The art of aging with grace, self-assurance, and a profound

appreciation for the beauty of experience are all part of your journey toward regeneration.

So, my reader, let's travel down this road together, where age is no barrier to beauty and where your journey through menopause and beyond is celebrated.

May you enjoy taking care of yourself and learn that true beauty comes from within, no matter how much time has passed.

CHAPTER ELEVEN
Rebirth and Renewal from Midlife to Second Spring

Imagine yourself at the beginning of a new season, where the potential of the present and the lessons of the past have merged.

Menopause is a shift that heralds a deep new beginning rather than an end. This chapter will discuss how your second spring might be defined by rebirth and regeneration.

The metaphor of the second spring

An old metaphor for menopause is a "second spring." Menopause can signal the beginning of a bright new stage of life—a period of rediscovery, self-renewal, and transformation—just as spring provides the promise of renewal and development after the dormancy of winter.

Accepting Change

It's imperative to accept the changes that menopause brings about to start on this journey of rebirth and regeneration.

It's time to let go of old habits and convictions that don't serve you anymore. You can get rid of everything that doesn't align with your actual essence, just like how trees shed their leaves in the fall.

The Knowledge of Experience

The wisdom of experience is most prominent during the menopause. Your life experiences have given you wisdom, fortitude, and a profound awareness of who you are.

The chances and challenges of this era can be successfully navigated with the help of this insight.

Finding Passion Again
Many women report that menopause gives them newfound vigor for living. There is more room to pursue your passions and ambitions when there are fewer external obligations.

It's a chance to pursue interests, hobbies, and adventures that may have been delayed.

Identity Reinvention
You can discover that your identity changes as you enter your second spring. You have the opportunity to reevaluate who you are and what you want at this stage of your life.

You are a dynamic, complex person who is not only characterized by your age or menopausal status.

Self-care should be prioritized.
Self-care becomes even more crucial after menopause. As you set out on this path of rebirth and regeneration, it's a way to take care of your body, mind, and spirit.

Make self-care a daily practice and let it sustain you throughout your second spring.

The Strength of Connection

Your journey to rebirth and rejuvenation depends critically on community and connection. Tell others about your experiences, stories, and observations.

Look for friends or support groups of like-minded people who are also going through this transformational period.

Your Particular Second Spring
Your second spring is wholly yours; it's a blank canvas that you may decorate with the vivid hues of rebirth and regeneration.

It's time to embrace your true self, rekindle your passions, and realize your full potential.

Remember that this is not the end of your adventure but rather a great new beginning as you begin this chapter.

Your second spring is a beautiful time to transform and flourish, and menopause is your invitation to do just that.

So let's start along this route together, dear reader, where menopause is not the goal but rather a stepping stone to a life of rejuvenation, meaning, and vigorous self-expression.

May this second spring, as you embrace the entirety of your journey to rebirth, be a time of tremendous development, joy, and self-discovery.

CHAPTER TWELVE
Wise Women's Wisdom: Stories of Triumph and Transformation

Imagine yourself beside a cozy fire, surrounded by learned women who have survived menopause to become sources of knowledge and inspiration. In this chapter, we'll discuss the experiences of women who overcame menopause and underwent significant change—women who were able to tap into their inner fortitude and appreciate the beauty of rebirth.

The Influence of Shared Stories

We have covered many aspects of menopause in this book, including its difficulties, mystique, and promise for rejuvenation.

It's time to hear from the women who have already traveled this route, from those who have weathered storms and discovered rainbows.

Triumphant Stories

Introducing Jane, a lady who used menopause as a chance to focus on self-care. She talks about how mindful exercise and cultivating self-love helped her regain her body.

The tale of Jane serves as a reminder that menopause is not the end but rather an opportunity for significant change.

Sarah is another; she became creative after going through menopause.

She shares the story of how she discovered her artistic abilities and used them to transform her feelings and fresh insight into stunning works of art.

A testament to the creative potential that can emerge from the depths of menopause is Sarah's narrative.

Transformational Stories

Lena's story illustrates how mindfulness may lead to transformation. She discusses how embracing mindfulness techniques helped her overcome crippling anxiety and restless nights.

Lena's story serves as a reminder that menopause can be a springboard for emotional fortitude and self-discovery.

Maria is another; she discovered her voice during menopause. She uses her newfound knowledge to inspire other women going through this phase by sharing her story of transitioning into advocacy.

The potential for menopause to spark a love for activism and community is highlighted by Maria's tale.

Common Wisdom

The menopause weaves a vast tapestry of experiences, and these women's stories are just a small part of it. They serve as a reminder that the menopause experience is varied and full of successes, changes, and newfound meaning.

Your Story

Think about your personal experience going through menopause as you read these stories. What victories and changes have you witnessed or hope to experience? Your experience is special and priceless, and it too might encourage others on their path to regeneration.

A Group of Wise Women

As we draw to a close, keep in mind that you belong to a group of knowledgeable women who have traveled this route. You are not alone in going through menopause; your experience proves your grit, fortitude, and the allure of rebirth.

So let's honor these great ladies and their tales of victory and transformation, dear reader. May their achievements and transformations serve as an example for you as you continue through menopause and give you the courage to embrace your own.

On this transforming journey, your narrative serves as a beacon of knowledge and hope for others, illuminating the path to rebirth for all women.